MDMA AND OTHER PSYCHEDELIC DRUGS

LEARNING THE THERAPEUTIC EFFECTS OF LSD, PSILOCYBIN AND OTHER MIND-BENDING DRUGS

BY SMART READS

Free Audiobook

As a thank you for being a Smart Reader you can choose 2 FREE audiobooks from audible.com. Simply sign up for free by visiting www.audibletrial.com/Travis to get your books.

Visit:

www.smartreads.co/freebooks
to receive Smart Reads books for FREE

Check us out on Instagram:

www.instagram.com/smart_readers
@smart_readers

ABOUT SMARTREADS

Choose Smart Reads and get smart every time. Smart Reads sorts through all the best content and condenses the most helpful information into easily digestible chunks.

We design our books to be short, easy to read and highly informative. Leaving you with maximum understanding in the least amount of time.

Smart Reads aims to accelerate the spread of quality information so we've taken the copyright off everything we publish and donate our material directly to the public domain. You can read our uncopyright below.

We believe in paying it forward and donate 5% of our net sales to Pencils of Promise to build schools, train teachers and support child education.

To limit our footprint and restore forests around the globe we are planting a tree for every 10 hardcover books we sell.

Thanks for choosing Smart Reads and helping us help the planet.

Sincerely,

Travis & the Smart Reads Team

Uncopyright 2017 by Smart Reads. No rights reserved worldwide. Any part of this publication may be reproduced or transmitted in any form without the prior written consent of the publisher.

Disclaimer: The publisher and author make no representations or warranties with respect to the accuracy or completeness of these contents and disclaim all warranties for a particular purpose. The author or publisher is not responsible for how you use this information. The fact that an individual or organization is referred to in this document as a citation or source of information does not imply that the author or publisher endorses the information that the individual or organization provided.

TABLE OF CONTENTS

Disclaimer:

This book and the information contained herein are in no way intended as an alternative to any medical advice. Individuals must take full responsibility and ensure that they obtain information from a trained health professional for any mental, physical or emotional health concerns.

INTRODUCTION

Originating from the Greek words: "psyche" which means soul or mind, and "delein" which means, "to manifest," the actual meaning of the word is psychedelic is "soul-manifesting." This implies that psychedelics provide access to the deepest parts of the soul and can develop unused potential of the human mind.

Psychedelic drugs are not the same as those drugs that would include opioids and stimulants. Those types of drugs produce states of altered consciousness whereas psychedelics affect the mind in a manner that is qualitatively different from those of usual consciousness.

In this modern world, the word "drugs" has become synonymous with many images and aspects, including addicts and dealers of all kinds. In this way it does have negative connotations attached to it. Psychedelic drugs, in particular, conjure up more images in people's minds, particularly of the 60's and 70's and more recently, of hard and dangerous party drugs, not to mention the issues of legality or rather, illegality, as many psychedelic drugs are illegal worldwide under UN conventions, unless they have some sort of medical or religious importance.

Many people who think about users of psychedelic drugs will often think about the high, or the visual or auditory hallucinations that are associated with them. A psychedelic drug is a medication whose primary action is to alter the individual's perception and cognition. Those individuals who take them seem to be more relaxed and happy. The question is: Is this actually the case? Are they happier?

According to a recent study whose findings were published in the Journal of Psychopharmacology, the answer would be yes. Non-psychedelic illicit drugs like cocaine and heroin are (rightly) associated with a lot of physical and psychological distress, including suicide. However, the information now being discovered about psychedelic drugs seems to be the opposite.

Science is now making some interesting discoveries about certain substances including ones that, for a long time have been considered to be Schedule 1 drugs. These are drugs that are considered dangerous, with a potential for abuse and with no medical value. Psychedelic drugs are still categorized as Schedule 1 along with other substances. This is one of the reasons it has been difficult to get funding for research over the past few decades, and therefore studies initiated decades earlier were never fully concluded.

Cannabis is one of the best known substances making a big splash in the medical world recently. The healing potential of certain strains of cannabis is being researched more and more and the results coming from this research and also clinical trials are showing that the potential is real and that more attention and funding must be given.

Anticipation has been mounting that in the U.S., the DEA (Drug Enforcement Agency) will make a decision about moving marijuana from a Schedule 1 to a Schedule II category. This regulatory move would free its use as a medicine for people suffering certain illnesses. The Agency still has not done this, however, and cannabis remains under the Schedule 1 category. This is even after so many studies and clinical trials that have clearly shown that cannabis does indeed have medicinal potential. This indicates that substances such as MDMA would then also not be moved from the Schedule 1 to the Schedule 2 category any time soon.

The FDA, however, has now approved several clinical trials on psychedelic drugs after a long period of prohibition in the United States. Substances such as

MDMA, LSD, and psilocybin are beginning to garner more attention. They are being investigated for their potential use in the treatment of certain mental conditions, such as depression.

So many individuals are suffering from a mental illness of some kind. Depression is one of the biggest ones as is anxiety. Then there are many with PTSD and addictions that are suffering and looking for something to assist them with their treatment. People are trying many different things to help them gain some control over their conditions, from behavioral therapy, to yoga and meditation, to big pharma drugs. They are looking into every corner.

This book will discuss some of the alternatives, including certain psychedelic drugs that have been and are still considered to be Schedule 1 by the government of the United States. The information is taken from a range of different sources and readers are also encouraged to do their own research and discover even more details about whichever aspect of this book they find themselves more drawn to.

CHAPTER 1: MDMA

In most instances, drugs such as LSD, MDMA and even cannabis are considered to be hard drugs and therefore classified as Schedule 1 substances by the United States government. Schedule 1 means these particular substances are illegal due to their high abuse potential and the belief that they hold no medical potential or usage, and come with severe safety concerns.

In many places, including the United States, Schedule 1 drugs are substances such as heroin, cocaine, LSD, ecstasy and cannabis, although cannabis has been decriminalized in many countries, and in some countries it was never on a Schedule 1 drug list to begin with. As with cannabis, medical professionals and researchers are now looking into the potential benefits that might be derived from these other "hard drug" substances, or more specifically, psychedelic drugs, just as in the case of cannabis which has recently received a lot of attention due to the discovery that it has valuable healing potential.

Due to the continued war on drugs, and of course, this also has its merits for some substances, funding for studies into any legitimate uses for these drugs is hard to come by. Street use of these drugs has been around for a long time. However, it is important to understand that anything bought on the street has usually been affected by (or cut) using other toxic chemicals including hair spray and even glass in some cases, in order to make it heavier therefore making more profit. Suppliers and dealers do not care about the well being of the people who buy it and the end product itself is often dangerous.

More serious controlled studies are now beginning to make their way back. Cannabis, as an example, has had a bad reputation in the U.S. for many decades, despite its medicinal potential being known and used in other places around the world. Distinguished universities such as Johns Hopkins and NYU are now looking into and researching the potential clinical psychiatric uses for substances that have been seen as dangerous for a long time.

MDMA is one of those drugs. Not to be confused with MDA or EMDA or even 2,3-MDMA; Methylenedioxymethamphetamine or MDMA for short, is a psychoactive drug which is commonly known ecstasy (E). It has been primarily used as a recreational drug creating effects such as euphoria, empathy, and other heightened sensations. It can and does have adverse effects too. These would include memory lapses, addiction, paranoia, insomnia, grinding teeth, sweating, blurred vision and rapid heartbeat. Deaths have also been reported by users due to an increase in body temperature, which can also lead to dehydration, however, other substances also affected the individuals at the time.

MDMA was created all the way back in 1912 by Anton Kollisch. It was originally developed to stop abnormal bleeding. It was later studied again and again and by 1977 it began to be used for its effects in psychotherapy due to its relaxation potential.

In the 1970's, it was utilized to help improve psychotherapy sessions. It then became a popular street drug during the 1980's. Often, when bought on the street, it has been mixed with other substances like amphetamine or methamphetamine; therefore its constitution becomes altered. In 2014, it was still popular, with around 9-29 million people using recreational ecstasy.

Could psychedelic drugs, in particular MDMA and LSD, actually have answers to mental health healing? According to some sources, as of 2017, MDMA has no accepted medicinal uses and MDMA is generally illegal in most countries. However, the above question is still being asked and limited exceptions are being made for research.

Smaller trials and further research have already begun. Contrary to the often-held belief that these drugs are only for those seeking a good rave or only for hippie types, some psychedelic drugs can have valid clinical uses.

MDMA is now thought to have potential uses in treating severe post-traumatic stress disorder (PTSD) of the type, which is treatment resistant. In the United States in 2016, the FDA has approved phase 3 clinical trials of MDMA for PTSD in order to examine safety and effectiveness.

MDMA, or ecstasy, has long been thought of as the choice for rave parties, festivals and clubs. In these environments, MDMA's sensory effects, combined with the lighting and music, are synergistic with the drug due to MDMA's psychedelic amphetamine traits.

Once MDMA has been taken, the reported effects take place within 30-60 minutes and can last for around 3 hours or more. The short-term psychoactive effects are reported to include:

- A sense of euphoria
- Relaxation
- Reduced anxiety

- Increased self-confidence
- Feelings of community with other users
- Inner peace
- Altered sense of time
- Mild hallucinations
- Enhanced sensations, perception, sexuality

Adverse short-term effects include:
- Dehydration
- Increased heart rate
- Increased blood pressure
- Appetite loss
- Diarrhea
- Insomnia
- Nausea and vomiting
- Excessive sweating
- Lethargy
- Irritability
- Dangerous to fetuses
- At very high doses, MDMA has shown to produce brain lesions and therefore some form of brain damage.

Of course, these feelings will depend on the amount of MDMA that was taken, the setting, and the individual. When it is taken in solitude and in a quiet setting it can have the effect of higher communication abilities, increased concentration and lucidity, and higher aesthetic sensitivity to emotions and background.

MDMA is sometimes referred to as being an empathogenic because it produces effects of empathy. Some studies have shown it has powerful empathy producing effects. In higher doses, MDMA users showed something else: an increase of hedonism and arousal continuum.

In the book, Through the Gateway of the Heart, Sophia Adamson, with a 6 page forward by Ralph Metzner, outlines a series of subjective anecdotes on the empathogenic experiences undergone by 50 participants who were in therapy due to traumatizing events. These people gave first-hand accounts of their experiences as they were administered the drug. The participants reported that MDMA's powerful qualities helped them become more open and talkative. The result was more successful therapy sessions. In 1985, the practice was banned but some researchers still continued with their studies.

In the early 2000's, the Multidisciplinary Association of Psychedelic Studies based in California, began studies on MDMA again. These studies aimed to show its efficacy in the treatment of mental health disorders, in particular anxiety and PTSD. The research so far has shown a long-lasting clinical improvement of PTSD symptoms. In 2008, the Multidisciplinary Association for Psychedelic Studies released a statement: "We found that low doses of MDMA (between 50 and 75 mg) were both psychologically and physiologically safe for all the subjects." The Association is now being funded for further research into the role of MDMA in the treatment of Post-Traumatic Stress Disorder. The results are positive with around 80% of participants responding successfully to the drug.

The Journal of Psychopharmacology reported that, *"MDMA-assisted psychotherapy compared with the same psychotherapy with inactive placebo produced clinically and statistically significant improvements in PTSD symptoms as measured by standard symptom scales. This difference was immediate and was maintained throughout the time period. There were no drug-related serious adverse events and no evidence of impaired cognitive function."*

This is not that surprising considering the information mentioned above and that recreational users have also reported benefits such as long-term positive mood changes and an overall sense of emotional well-being. Considering the fact that mental illness is at endemic proportions today in our culture, these results are a positive step and will hopefully lead to more research and clinical trials. The question that arises is if the new anti-drug administration will allow the past studies and data to be accessed and whether they will then change the category of MDMA from a Schedule 1 drug to something lesser and allow it to be re-examined for its medical potential.

CHAPTER 2: MDMA AND PTSD

In November 2016, the New York Times reported that the drug ecstasy, or more precisely, its active ingredient 3,4-methylenedioxy-N-mthylamphetamine, (MDMA), is set to be studied in a large-scale clinical trial. Indeed, the FDA has approved a series of three trials of MDMA. The trials are intended for those suffering from PTSD, in particular the PTSD that cannot be treated with more established therapy. This is the final stage of validation that will change the image of MDMA from a party drug to a legal medicine with healing potential.

MDMA has already shown promise in its effectiveness in treating people with PTSD in some smaller studies sponsored by the Multidisciplinary Association for Psychedelic Studies (or MAPS). This organization advocates for medical research on certain psychedelic substances. The Drug Enforcement Administration currently still lists MDMA as a Schedule 1 substance. Incidentally, cannabis is also listed as a Schedule 1 substance and is now being legalized due to its medical potential being realized. If these trials on MDMA go well, it could be made legal by 2021.

So how does MDMA work on the human brain to help those suffering from PTSD?

Well, it has more than one effect on the human brain and it seems to assist the process of moving through past trauma in a more effective way. At this point, talk therapy or psychotherapy is how PTSD is treated, and in many people it doesn't work that well as an effective and long-term treatment. There are certain drugs that have been approved for PTSD treatment, but according to some doctors, they only target symptoms.

Researchers now believe MDMA has the potential to improve how patients with PTSD respond when undergoing psychotherapy. It seems to act as a type of catalyst for patients and helps them when talking through and processing their trauma. So it seems that MDMA helps to make the psychotherapy more effective and patients can move through memories and trauma more effectively.

MDMA creates a significant increase in neurotransmitter levels in the brain, in particular serotonin. This is a big contributor to creating a feeling of happiness and well-being. Serotonin also increases the levels of some hormones such as oxytocin, (sometimes referred to as the "love hormone" as it increases affiliative behavior and enables people to connect with others), and prolactin which can create a state of relaxation and satisfaction.

Oxytocin also affects how people respond to certain facial expressions. They are less likely to interpret them as angry or threatening and this can be crucial in psychotherapy because PTSD sufferers tend to be extra vigilant and are constantly looking for anything they might interpret as a threat.

Considering the effects that MDMA can have and the hormone levels it produces, it is not difficult to see how patients can benefit from it. People move into what is termed the "optimal arousal zone" while engaging in therapy. If those suffering from PTSD are over-aroused then they cannot engage in therapy and it won't work well for them. If they feel more relaxed and less threatened, then therapy can have more of a chance.

Patients given MDMA are more likely to use words that relate to support, intimacy and friendship. It seems to enhance the quality of their social interactions. This, in turn helps to improve relationships. It also enhances levels of shared empathy and social behavior. A recent test using a simulated paradigm of social exclusion conducted by

Frye et al. showed that participants who were given MDMA showed reduced social exclusion tendencies.

In other studies, such as Wardle et al., MDMA was shown to facilitate faster identification of happy faces. It also reduced the detection of negative or threatening facial expressions. This is significant when dealing with patients suffering severe PTSD.

One study done in South Carolina involving 20 patients who were mostly sexual abuse victims with PTSD, found that of those given the MDMA, 83% no longer met the criteria of PTSD after their treatment. That is compared to only 25% of those who were not given MDMA.

In the follow-up to this particular study, which was done almost 4 years later, the results that were discovered were pleasing indeed. The participants showed more improvement the further out they were from the MDMA assisted psychotherapy. This means that the provided treatment not only gave immediate relief, but a continued and sustained healing in the longer term.

It is important to understand that those with PTSD will not necessarily feel completely happy and relaxed when taking MDMA. Patients do tend to have positive experiences, however, they did not feel euphoric. Trauma is always painful and difficult to process, but MDMA seems to help patients feel like they can process their trauma without getting too overwhelmed.

There can side effects when using MDMA and it is important to mention this. Short-term side effects can include a decreasing appetite, jaw clenching, nausea, sweating, chills and high blood pressure. However, this drug is not going to be something available over the counter. It will be strictly controlled and therapists will administer it to patients in correct dosages and monitor them carefully throughout their treatment.

MDMA does not cause hallucinations, as can be the case with psilocybin. It elicits healing through different mechanisms, as mentioned above. Psychotherapists have actually used it since the 1970's as an underground adjuvant - a pharmacology drug or agent added to another drug or agent to enhance its medical effectiveness.

It is also important to mention that MDMA, or ecstasy available on the street are absolutely not the same thing. That which can be bought on the street is not pure and usually contains other dangerous chemicals and harmful adulterants. MDMA given to patients during trials is definitely pharmaceutical grade and is given at the right dosage by trained professionals. MDMA already has the reputation of making people feel more open and trusting wherever they may be – on the dance floor, at a music festival, etc. The party drug ecstasy is not likely to contain much MDMA, if it contains any at all. However, actual MDMA has shown some compelling results.

The optimal PTSD treatment would include strategies for calming the symptoms as well as careful re-examination and re-processing of the trauma triggers. Through MDMA psychotherapy, both of these can be achieved. This is because, when it is used together with psychotherapy, the MDMA drug helps patients to identify the actual root cause of their suffering and they can do this without becoming re-traumatized.

The serotonin that is produced through the help of MDMA will reduce fear and depression and allow patients to focus on their trauma in therapy sessions without triggering their sympathetic nervous systems. This will inhibit patients becoming overwhelmed by their negative feelings and thoughts.

It helps PTSD sufferers to think about things from a different angle. It therefore allows patients to begin making new connections and associations, and in this way it starts re-wiring the brain. The substances in MDMA not only allow patients to feel relaxed and calm but ensure they remain alert as well. It is this balance of attentiveness and relaxation that will contribute positively to the healing process.

Psychiatrist and psychopharmacologist, Julia Holland explains: "It's almost like anesthesia for surgery... It allows you to dig and get to the malignant thing that needs to be pulled out and examined. It takes years in psychotherapy to dig around the trauma and start to get to it. This is a way for people to process the core issue in order to move forward... You basically couldn't design a molecule that is better for therapy than MDMA."

Other medications such as benzodiazepines and SSRIs, which have traditionally been used to treat PTSD, only numb the unpleasant symptoms. MDMA allows those suffering from the debilitating PTSD to dig deeper into their own psyche in order to heal themselves.

One of the MAPS (Multidisciplinary Association for Psychedelic Studies) studies involved 19 women who were suffering from PTSD due to sexual assault. In that particular study, 83% of the women who received psychotherapy along with MDMA were not categorized as having PTSD after the treatment was over, according to Brad Burge who is the director of communications and marketing. The psychotherapy itself is actually very good, however, for some patients with treatment-resistant PTSD, MDMA is a big help and moves the therapy along faster and better.

Of course, not everyone or anyone will be able to administer MDMA psychotherapy. There is a strict certification process that must be put into place for professional and licensed therapists who might want to use MDMA.

Another question to ask is whether or not there are any effects when people are coming off MDMA. Well, at this stage there doesn't seem to be any issues. Researchers so far have found that, even though MDMA causes the brain to release certain chemicals such as oxytocin and serotonin, psychotherapists can alleviate some of those effects that might arise from the depletion. There were some earlier studies, which concluded that MDMA might not be side effect free. These were done by the National Institute of Drug Abuse and concluded that there could be long-term damage to serotonin containing neurons and the brain itself. These findings have now been seriously challenged by more recent independent studies.

It is necessary to understand that MDMA does not make people become completely "blissed out" and then they are cured and fine. It is a lot of hard work and also still painful but MDMA makes it possible. It acts as a catalyst to the process and continues to unfold for weeks or even the rest of someone's life. This means that MDMA is not the actual cure as such, but a powerful and effective catalyst for the psychotherapy.

So, what is the future of MDMA?

It is possible that a few years from now, doctors could be prescribing MDMA to help with post-traumatic stress disorder. Perhaps a few years more, and it might even be prescribed for anxiety.

Since the Multidisciplinary Association for Psychedelic Studies is in the process of wrapping up the second phase of the FDA clinical trials on MDMA-assisted PTSD psychotherapy, phase 3 will soon begin. This means that the U.S. government could issue a decision on the drug's usage as early as 2021.

If the FDA approves MDMA use for cases of PTSD related psychotherapy, MAPS is hopeful that this will encourage that it also be used for certain other cases as well. Already, MDMA psychotherapy is being explored with patients who suffer from severe anxiety due to life-threatening illnesses such as cancer.

In addition, using MDMA as a possible tool for autistic adults is being looked into. This would include helping them with social skills. As mentioned, the phase 3 trials will begin and FDA approval must be given before any of this can take place. However, since the research so far is showing such positive results, it is likely that MDMA-assisted psychotherapy could become more prominent in the not so distant future.

CHAPTER 3: PSILOCYBIN

Psilocybin, otherwise known by its more popular name "magic mushrooms," is a naturally occurring psychoactive ingredient. It has been a favorite hallucinogen for illicit users for many years. At first glance, these little white and brown mushrooms don't seem to be particularly magical, but those who have tried a dose of it swear by its life-changing potential.

These mushrooms come in about 100 different species that contain compounds known as psilocybin and psilocin. They are psychoactive and can cause hallucinations as well as euphoria and other existential symptoms. They have been used in Central America well before Europeans landed on their shores, in religious and/or spiritual ceremonies. In the U.S., they are part of the black market drug trade and are considered an illegal substance.

The compounds in psilocybin mushrooms give users a "mind-melting" type of feeling, but in fact, the opposite is true. Psilocybin actually boosts the brain's connectivity allowing it to synchronize activity among areas that would not normally be connected. They have also been shown to slow down activity in information-transfer areas of the brain like the thalmus. This slowing down allows information to travel more freely through the brain. A dose of psilocybin can alter an individual's personality, making them more open to new experiences. People who have more open personalities tend to be more creative, more appreciative, and more emotionally available. The substance does indeed have effects on emotions with people reporting profound experiences including feelings of full joy and connectedness to others.

Psilocybin is known to promote a sense of well-being and calm. It has been tested recently on patients with advanced stages of cancer to control depression and anxiety. The FDA gave the all clear for the study, which was led by Charles S. Grob M.D. at UCLA. The aim was to find out if there could be any clinical benefits for the patients.

With this first study, it was discovered after close monitoring of the patients, that they reported a noticeable decrease in anxiety, depression and fear that lasted up to six months after just one dose. This has led to more studies being done on psilocybin at NYU, Johns Hopkins and the University of Alabama. The studies embarked upon in those places have shown similar results.

Psilocybin is being studied more and more for its potentially healing role in the treatment of anxiety and depression. It is a naturally occurring alkaloid. It is considered to be a recreational substance, however, recent population based studies show that it doesn't lead to serious mental or physical problems. This would include dependence.

Psilocybin has a psychopharmacological action believed to be mediated through binding to serotonergic 5-HT receptors, among others. This in turn will provide anti-anxiety and antidepressant effects. It is a lot more complicated than what has been described above, however, this book is intended to be written in as simple a format as possible.

In a recent study, researchers attempted to discover psilocybin's potential, safety and effectiveness when used on people with treatment-resistant unipolar depression. This is a brain disorder that sees people remain in a persistently depressed state with little or no interest in activities. It can have a significant impairment on daily life.

In the first instance, psilocybin was administered to the patients with psychological support included, of course. Patients who suffered from moderate to severe unipolar depression and who were unresponsive to more than two antidepressants that were administered were tested using psilocybin. They were given low doses (10 mg) of oral psilocybin initially, and then another higher dose of 25 mg one week later. It was found that the psilocybin was well tolerated by all the patients tested and there were no unexpected or serious adverse effects.

It was found that the depressive symptoms of patients were significantly reduced, first of all at the one week mark, and then again after three months of treatment. After the study was done, it was clear that there is therapeutic potential and it would be wise to conduct more rigorous studies in order to investigate its potential even further.

The most important requirement of a pharmacological agent, which is to be utilized as a medicinal drug, is that it must be adequately safe when it is administered to people. In the abovementioned study, the psilocybin doses that were used were found to be safe when given to people who were healthy and people who had medical and/or psychiatric illnesses.

Another study conducted on 36 healthy people who were given 30 mg of psilocybin, found that there was no persistent harmful psychological or physiological effects. In another instance, researchers explored psilocybin's effects on anxiety on people with advanced cancer, it was found that there were no clinically adverse effects.

Secondly, in order for a psychedelic drug to be viably used as a pharmacological agent, the acute effects must be easy to manage and well tolerated. Psilocybin has been found to produce mild and pleasurable effects that are non-threatening in a trial conducted on 110 individuals. It therefore seems that evidence is growing which shows that a neurological basis for psilocybin's efficacy in the treatment of unipolar depression has much potential.

Using functional magnetic resonance imaging, or fMRI scans; it was found that psilocybin de-activated the medial prefrontal cortex. It found that those suffering from depression have a hyperactive medial prefrontal cortex and with effective treatment this hyperactivity is normalized. Therefore, psilocybin's consistency in its effectiveness in depression treatment cannot be ignored.

Other fMRI studies have shown that the amygdala activation decreases with the use of psilocybin. It decreases the response to threat-related visual stimuli. It also decreases threat-induced modulation of top-down connectivity from the amygdala to the primary visual cortex. Both these mechanisms tend to produce positive affect states. The amygdala has a key role in the perception and generation of emotions. It can become hyperactive in response to negative stimuli and this in turn leads to negative moods in patients who are depressed.

Many therapists believe that anxiety, depression and OCD (obsessive compulsive disorder) are likely the result of a hyperactive default network within certain areas of the brain. In patients who suffer from depression, the brain's network patterns are of self-depreciating thoughts. They might go something like this: I can't make it, I'm a loser, nothing goes my way…. etc. etc. When using therapy in conjunction with psilocybin this default network decreases the hyperactive activity and the separation between the resting state network of the brain decreases significantly. It allows for the breaking of harmful patterns and lets the brain make new connections. This seems to be how psychedelics improve mental health.

With regards to cancer patients, they already have a lot to deal with. Cancer is a brutal disease and takes a toll not only on the body but also on the mind. The emotional toll can be exceptionally difficult. Cancer patients have levels of depression and anxiety, which tend to be quite high and difficult to bear. Even those in remission continue to suffer from depression and anxiety.

Two studies which were released simultaneously by researchers at Johns Hopkins and New York University show that just one dose of psilocybin can actually ease both anxiety and depression for up to six months. This is indeed a very promising result and has great potential for those dealing with cancer and the fear that comes with it. In many of these cases, patients do not respond to traditional psychotherapy or antidepressants.

Both studies were published in the Journal of Psychpharmacology. They were accompanied by eleven editorials of support from leading figures in psychiatry as well as two former American Psychiatric Association presidents. Dr. Stephen Ross, director of substance abuse services in the Department of Psychiatry at NYU stated, "Our results represent the strongest evidence to date of a clinical benefit from psilocybin therapy, with the potential to transform care for patients with cancer-related psychological distress."

The study conducted at NYU involved 29 individuals who were suffering serious psychological distress, which stemmed from advanced stages of cancer. Some of these people were in remission. Every person received a capsule of psilocybin or a placebo capsule. In the second session they were given the opposite, i.e. those that took the psilocybin took the placebo and those who took the placebo were given the psilocybin. The sessions were between four to six hours long. The results were quite impressive. Between 60-80% of patients reported a reduction in anxiety and depression. This lasted up to six months after they were given the treatment.

At Johns Hopkins, the study included 51 individuals and the results were similar. The patients received one dose of psilocybin. Six months later, 80% of the individuals in the trial continued to show a decrease in anxiety and depression. Meanwhile, 83% reported an increase in life satisfaction and well-being. Furthermore, 67% of participants stated that the trial was in the top five most meaningful experiences they'd had in their lives. Some of the participants stated that they experienced a feeling of overwhelming love and felt immediately changed.

One patient who had severe anxiety about ovarian cancer recurring, stated, "My fear and anxiety were completely removed, and they haven't come back." The wife of another participant whose husband had cancer and eventually died from the illness stated that her husband was "reborn into this place of personal and universal love. He said he felt it all around him, and he felt a sense of forgiveness too."

The Berkley Foundation, particularly the Berckley/Imperial Psychedelic Research Programme, had a particularly good year in 2016. In May, it published the first results from psilocybin's effect on people with treatment-resistant depression. Results were promising with most participants experiencing immediate and sustained improvement of depressive symptoms, and 42% remaining depression free at the three-month follow-up. In fact, just one psilocybin dose outperformed sustained courses of more traditional medication and psychotherapy up to three months after the initial dosage was given.

Brain-imaging studies have shown that psilocybin produces a global increase in the cerebral metabolic glucose rate, in particular of the frontal-medial and frontolateral cortex. These changes will affect the psychological state of the individual. When psilocybin is administered correctly and under the supervision of a trained professional, there have been no sustained detrimental psychological or physiological effects. Not only that, but there is also evidence that it can have significantly lasting improvements on the individuals' quality of life.

Psilocybin and other psychedelic drugs have been recognized for many years as potential therapeutic agents. However, the strict drug laws in the U.S. stalled the research. It was really when the drugs started to be used more and more as recreational drugs that it became quite a cause for concern. This overshadowed the possible therapeutic benefits. Psychedelic drugs, including psilocybin, were then classified as Schedule 1 drugs. This meant that the U.S. government now considered it to have a high potential for abuse. This made any continued research almost impossible even though experts had stated at the time that negative side-effects (such as nausea and headaches) were rare when administered responsibly.

Dr. Ross says he could not understand how something of such significance had been buried. The restriction meant that even today, it took about two years for the hospital to get the go-ahead for their research. Despite the positive results, there is still a concern that the pharmaceutical companies won't see any financial incentive in a drug that only needs a single dose. This could impact on psilocybin being made available as a therapeutic drug.

As mentioned already, some psychedelic drugs have already been used in the past to assist in psychotherapy. A neurological basis for them to be utilized is now emerging as well. Psilocybin has been found to strongly facilitate the activation of certain areas of the brain. These would include the limbic system that responds to autobiographical memory prompts. This salient memory facilitation during psychotherapy can be significant.

What is the future of psylocybin?

In recent years, awareness has been growing about the psychological and spiritual experiences people receive when administered with certain psychedelics, psilocybin being one of them. There has also been a growing awareness of what cancer patients, and others with terminal illnesses, as well as their loved ones experience. These need to be addressed even more than they have been in the past.

Although current evidence of psilocybin's potential is limited, what evidence there is does indeed suggest that it can possibly be a safe, effective and feasible pharmacological agent in the treatment of depression. The most recent clinical studies of psilocybin show that it is not harmful to human physical or psychological health. At this stage, however, it seems to be limited to patients who have shown a resistance to, or are not responding to conventional therapy treatment. More research and clinical trials are needed and researchers remain hopeful that this will occur in the near future.

CHAPTER 4: LSD

LSD, or lysergic acid diethylamide, was actually created in 1938 in Switzerland by Albert Hoffman. LSD was developed at the Sandoz pharmaceutical company in Basel, Switzerland and is actually a partially synthetic compound. In 1943, Dr. Hoffman found its promising effects and it was quickly recognized for the potential therapeutic effects it could have. In addition, LSD played a major role in the discovery of the serotonin neurotransmitter system.

With the mention of LSD, it often brings up images of the 60's and 70's and the hippie era. It is well known for its ability to bring on mystical or spiritual experiences and to facilitate strong feelings of connectedness. However, as mentioned above, it was originally considered a promising psychiatric drug when it was first created. Numerous studies were performed to test for LSD's efficacy in treating various mental health conditions. Unfortunately, any funding that may have been forthcoming was cut swiftly in the U.S. after it was listed by the DEA as a Schedule 1 drug in 1967.

LSD has also had some positive results from testing done in alcohol addiction treatment facilities from the 50's to the 70's. Therapists, psychiatrists, and researchers would administer LSD to literally thousands of individuals. This was done to treat anxiety, depression, and alcoholism.

More studies are now being planned to get a better idea of the true efficacy, and now, after a forty year pause on medical research, the Food and Drug Administration's first LSD approved study results will finally be released, bringing this drug's potential medicinal benefits into the spotlight.

Scientists began to pick up where, in the 1960's before the ban, the medical community left off. They recently began investigating LSD's effects when combined with therapy on twelve terminally ill individuals. The results from that controlled study have been published in the peer-reviewed Journal of Nervous and Mental Disease. They showed that when LSD was combined with psychotherapy, it significantly eased anxiety about the end of life for patients suffering terminal illnesses.

The twelve patients were separated into two groups and they both had to undergo two preparatory sessions before any LSD was administered. The participants had to cease any and all antidepressant and/or anti-anxiety medication they were taking.

They were also asked to avoid alcohol a day before the study.

One of the groups was given 200 micrograms of LSD. The other was given 20 micrograms, which is minimal. Every participant had two dosing sessions, each a few weeks apart. Of course, therapists assisted and would walk them through their individual experiences with the help of the psychedelics they were taking. Those who were given the 200 micrograms were found not to have any long-term negative side effects from the drug. This is what was reported by the participants.

They reported a lessening of their anxiety and depression. Not only was this reported during the sessions and immediately after, but it was the same situation that was maintained in the longer-term. The individuals who were only administered 20 micrograms, on the other hand, reported an increase in their anxiety levels.

This study was able to take place because, as Rick Doblin, founder of MAPS stated, "People are more scared of dying than they are of using drugs. That's why we were able to start LSD research with people who were anxious about dying, that and the combination of Albert Hoffman and good contacts with the Swiss equivalent of the FDA."

Psychotherapist and author of the book Psychedelic
Healing, Neal M. Goldsmith explained the importance
of the research. He said that it has long-term
implications for society as a whole. It will help people
in the short-term as well, and the real question is:
what is the benefit of relaxation, relief or spiritual
epiphany? It is also a question of what the effects are
on people who are dying. He believes that society will
become better once psychedelics are reintegrated
because society will be changed as it creates changes
in itself.

There is still a way to go to discover more about
exactly how LSD works on the brain. However, Doblin
mentioned what they know so far about how it works
is that its psychoactive ingredients will interact with
the filtering system of the brain. This will allow those
thoughts and feelings that are deeply suppressed to be
revealed, and this will then make the way for a
"confrontation" so to speak, and the potential for
healing.

Breaking harmful neural patterns and letting the brain
make new connections is one way in which
psychedelics work to improve mental health. In 2016,
Carhart-Harris, a neuropsychopharmacologist,
scanned 20 healthy volunteers' brains during a 6-hour

LSD session. The scans were then compared to the control volunteers, and showed a noticeable decrease in the default-mode network, which is a brain area responsible for automatic, mindless background thinking. For people suffering with depression, for example, this background thinking is continually saying negative things that distract from life in general. To be able to slow this down or reduce it significantly will help those suffering depression or anxiety.

In trials conducted on both LSD and psilocybin, there were no flashbacks, psychosis, or other serious adverse symptoms. What was significant was the intensity of the spiritual or mystical experiences described by the participants.

These spiritual experiences were noted in other studies as well. For example, a recent study was done on 15 smokers who received psilocybin for CBT – cognitive behavioral therapy. From the 15 individuals, 80% of them showed that even at the 6-month follow-up they remained smoke free. At the 12-month follow-up the majority – 67% were still smoke-free.

This phenomenon can likely explain the efficacy of LSD in helping to reduce alcohol addiction.

More recently, the Berkley Foundation completed an important brain-imaging study, which was intended to discover more information on the effects that LSD can have on humans. The results were published in the prestigious journal PNAS, (Proceedings of the National Academy of Sciences of the United States of America). It is the scientific journal of the National Academy of Sciences and has been published since 1915.The brain-imaging clearly displayed how the dominance of particular brain-networks - like the controlling default-mode network which is currently described as the neural relation of the ego, is significantly lessened under the effects of LSD. Not only that, but communication between other networks is significantly expanded.

Some understanding of how the blood supply and neuronal activity works will help to explain how psychedelics affect us and also how they can actually be such powerful medicine. The observations so far have been that underlying similarities in behavior such as anxiety, depression, OCD, and addiction, is quite a rigidly set pattern of thoughts. Drugs such as psychedelics seem to be able to rattle this rigidity and allow a window to open up which in turn allows for therapeutic intervention that can replace the damaging behavioral patterns and replace them with more flexible and positive ones.

Despite all this research and the positive results that are stemming from it, LSD is still not legally allowed to be used on patients. Not only does this apply to the U.S. but to many other nations as well. However, there is one doctor who is legally allowed to use LSD in his practice and on his patients by his government.

Dr. Peter Gasser is a Swiss psychiatrist and has spent almost a decade delving into psychedelic research. He picked up pretty much where Albert Hoffman left off in 1966. If you recall, Hoffman was the first to synthesize and ingest LSD then record his experiences. Dr. Hoffman met with Gasser personally on a number of occasions and gave him his approval to move further into experimental therapy assisted by drugs of a psychedelic nature.

Gasser, who took LSD about 25 years ago, has been interested in psychedelics from a medicinal viewpoint. In 1988, the Swiss Federal Office for Public Health to start research using LSD granted him permission. This was despite the global ban on the drug. Gasser was one of only five therapists in Switzerland legally permitted to implement both LSD and MDMA into his research. He was also legally permitted to try the psychoactive treatment himself until LSD was banned in 1993.

Despite the ban, Gasser didn't stop integrating LSD into his therapy research. His stance was that, since these substances are a reality, it is more helpful to fully investigate potential benefits as well as potential risks than to prevent banned substances being used underground and in potentially destructive ways.

Fast forward a couple of decades, and the Swiss Ministry of Health approved Gassers' pilot study that delved into LSD's effects when administered to patients who are suffering from terminal illnesses such as cancer, among others. This study was sponsored by MAPS.

This study included every patient undergoing two drug assisted therapy sessions. There was a short break in between them. The findings were finally published after seven years of research. This was the first controlled trial of LSD in the 21st Century. It was published under the name: "LSD-assisted psychotherapy for anxiety associated with a life-threatening disease: A qualitative study of acute and sustained subjective effects."

Some of the participants died in the first year of the trial, however, they did have the chance to have their anxiety, depression, and gloom eased significantly in their remaining days.

Gasser was also asked to speak at Horizons: Perspectives in Psychedelic Research, which held a conference in New York City. There, he presented data from his pilot study. He explained that he had successfully campaigned the Swiss government to allow him "compassionate use" and include LSD in his therapeutic practice. Gasser still administers LSD to his patients, in group as well as individual settings. Another Swiss doctor who works not far from Gasser has permission from the government to work with MDMA in the same way.

Gasser is convinced that LSD brings additional benefits for patients. He bases this not only on his extensive studies with patients, but also on his own experiences when he was using it himself when he was younger. He believes that LSD should have its place among the many other methods of treating patients and that it is not the only one or the best one. He mentions, however, that for some people it is very helpful to be able to move into an altered mind state and to have spiritual or mystic experiences - things that cannot really be achieved through standard therapy.

Gasser worked with cancer patients during his study. His thinking was that an individual with a life-threatening illness is much confronted with issues of an existential nature and must deal with a lot of anxiety.

When it comes to the issue of dosing and frequency of use, Gasser stated that he is allowed to give as much as 200 micrograms in one therapy session, the same as what he gave while doing the study. However, he often gives only 100 micrograms when administering it to a patient for the first time as he feels it's enough and it often works better. A high dosage may frighten the individual, or if it's too high the person may not actually relax but be more stressed. He carefully analyzes the patient and the situation and decides what dosage to give.

Gasser is quick to ensure that people understand that simply taking LSD will not just make everything fantastic and make all their problems go away. Difficult times will still be there but working through them with a therapist or some sort of guide who can assist them to embrace or integrate the difficult experiences is necessary.
Using LSD in therapy is not only for terminally-ill patients, however. Gasser has also used this therapy with others and gives some examples of patients'

issues to show how LSD can help. There are also other situations in life when individuals are faced with some deep and important issues that LSD might help with. Gasser is careful to ask himself what medical condition LSD can assist with and which ones it cannot.

He spoke about a young many who was doing his PhD and was suffering from severe anxiety disorder. This caused him to experience debilitating stress if he had to speak at a seminar or during group tasks. He had undergone a lot of treatment already, including psychological, medical and Jungian psychoanalysis. All these helped him only to a certain degree but he could not move through his social anxiety in a controlled setting.

He finally approached Gasser who told him to try the LSD in group therapy (the groups are small – only three people) that he was organizing. He was able to get the Swiss government to agree to group LSD therapy, but it wasn't easy. The young man was frightened by this concept initially, but after his first small group therapy session, he emerged saying he had a fantastic experience and that for the first time he had not felt threatened by other people in a group setting. This was the first breakthrough for him. Now this individual will go ahead and try to bring this experience to his life in general and to his work and studies. He also stated that he didn't feel that he needed to have another session for a while.

What is the future of LSD?

LSD, like the other psychedelics mentioned in this book, has the potential to allow patients to delve deeper into their own minds and access areas that have been previously out of reach. Even though using LSD may seem puzzling to some professionals, the latest studies as well as the older ones, clearly show it is indeed a substance that needs to be taken more seriously as a therapeutic tool. It can definitely be used as a catalyst or an amplifier of the mental process.

LSD came into the scene at a time when the psychopharmacological field was experiencing a type of revolution. Tranquilizers, antidepressants etc., were having their initial triumphs at the time and creating a hope that an easy chemical solution for certain mental conditions could be found.

Since MAPS has already completed the first parts of its research, which it started in 2014, the results have been hailed as positive. Of course, this follows on the heels of the original studies done decades earlier, but they had to be stopped due to a lack of funding and legal issues. The MAPS study was viewed as a big success because there were not any noteworthy adverse effects. It was also considered successful due to the fact that all of the participants reported that they got personal benefits from the treatment and that those effects continued to remain stable over time.

With more new research continuing and more discoveries being made and explored, the future of LSD seems to indeed be promising as it relates to its application as a therapy. Unfortunately, it is still an illegal substance. However, this may change with the passing of time and more information becoming available.

CONCLUSION

MDMA, psilocybin, and LSD have proven that they, being psychedelic drugs mentioned in this book, are a powerful and unique tool to help humans explore human nature and the human mind. Psychedelic experiences have the ability to assist us in mediating the deeper realms of our psyche that have, for the most part, not been discovered or acknowledged by mainstream psychology and psychiatry. These drugs also reveal more possibilities, including different means to access therapeutic changes and personality transformations.

Of course, as with anything that is being experimented on for the first time, psychedelic experimentation could also have dangers and/or pitfalls. However, until this point the only side-effects seems to be mild, such as nausea and blood pressure, and they fade with the passing of only a little bit of time. Ventures into areas that have been unexplored will always carry some risk but the way that the research and testing has been done is ensuring minimal risks and maximum benefits to the patients.

The fact that cannabis laws have already been changed in many nations and are changing in the U.S. too is evidence that some sort of logic is being applied when it comes to testing and discovering potential medicinal uses for certain drugs. It is also important to remember that psychedelics were being used, in particular ancient cultures, and even some cultures today continue to use them without the stigma that exists in the U.S.

The fact that the psychedelic drugs discussed in this book are all classified as Schedule 1 substances and are totally banned is an impediment to the way research is being done and the way that it might continue to be done, or even if it continues at all. Funding is necessary and more funding will come only when the severe restrictions are lifted. There could be a wider spectrum of research undertaken and these substances could have their potential efficacy seriously considered in other unexplored healthcare areas.

This might include areas such as Alzheimer's research or studies done on the efficacy with dementia patients. Full clinical trials could also be conducted. These are necessary to demonstrate beyond any doubt that these substances do indeed have therapeutic value. The way would then be paved for them to be developed into medicines that could be actually life changing.

It is not only about changing the restrictions on scheduled drugs, but also about changing the public perception on psychedelic drugs. More often than not, this perception is dominated by skepticism and fear. Of course, this has come about due to entire generations being told over and over about how harmful, toxic and/or dangerous these drugs are. Any type of substance can be misused and can cause harm when administered wrongly, but these problems will not be corrected by banning the substances completely. Scheduling laws, which prevent even the most basic research that could reveal not only their therapeutic value, but also any potential harmful effects, if there are any, also cannot solve them. Many drugs are prescribed responsibly and used responsibly by doctors and patients alike. There are also many drugs that have the potential to be abused and misused, and they are.

One example would be amphetamines. They are being prescribed as a treatment for things like ADHD (attention deficit hyperactivity disorder). They are also taken as a stimulant. Another example would be opiates, which would include substances such as morphine and heroin. Morphine has long been used as a painkiller. Heroin does not seem to have therapeutic benefits at this stage and is indeed highly addictive. It's important to start looking at psychedelics in the same way - to look at them with clinical oversight, to explore their therapeutic benefits and also check for any risks.

Today, everything is moving rapidly and where attitudes can change just as rapidly. There is a lot of hope for the future despite so many negatives in the world. It is highly likely that more and more there will be some amazing breakthroughs and scientific research will become wider and more encompassing.

With more sufficient funding, research into many areas, not only limited to the therapeutic potential of psychedelic drugs, could be and should be expanded. This could make a huge difference to treatment-resistant conditions such as PTSD, OCD, and addictions, as well as assisting depression and anxiety, especially in those with life-threatening illnesses.

Psychedelics could also be used to enhance creativity, neuroplasticity as well as general well being. It is hopeful that the groundbreaking scientific research already mentioned in this book, and other research still going on, will start the ball rolling on reform when it comes to prohibitive policies, and will create a safe space where people can access what they need and whatever will assist them to attain a state of physical or mental health.

It is indeed an exciting time in psychedelic research. Medical researchers are getting the go-ahead to delve further into the potential these drugs can have on humans and the trials that have already been conducted are promising. This leads to the conclusion that future research will likely be funded and just as likely the results will be positive. The stigma around psychedelic drugs is beginning to shift and even journalists are not worried about discussing their therapeutic potential.

THANKS FOR READING

We really hope you enjoyed this book. If you found this material helpful feel free to share it with friends. You can also help others find it by leaving a review where you purchased the book. Your feedback will help us continue to write books you love.

The Smart Reads library is growing by the day! Make sure and check out the other wonderful books in our catalog. We would love to hear which books are your favorite.

SMART READS ORIGINS

Smart Reads was born out of the desire to find the best information fast without having to wade through the sheer volume of fluff available online. Smart Reads combs through massive amounts of knowledge compiles the best into quick to read books on a variety of subjects.

We consider ourselves Smart Readers, not dummies. We know reading is smart. We're self taught. We like to learn a TON about a WIDE variety of topics. We have developed a love for books and we find intelligence attractive.

We found that each new topic we tried to learn about started with the challenge of finding the pieces of the puzzle that mattered most. It becomes a treasure hunt rather than an education.

Smart Reads wants to find the best of the best information for you. To condense it into a package that you can consume in an hour or less. So you can read more books about more topics in less time.

OUR MISSION

Smart Reads aims to accelerate the availability of useful information and will publish a high quality book on every major topic on amazon.

Smart Reads hopes to remove barriers to sharing by taking the copyright off everything we publish and donating it to the public domain. We hope other publishers and authors will follow our example.

Our goal is to donate $1,000,000 or more by 2020 to build over 2,000 schools by giving 5% of our net profit to Pencils of Promise.

We want to restore forests around the globe by planting a tree for every 10 physical books we sell and hope to plant over 100,000 trees by 2020.

Doesn't it feel good knowing that by educating yourself you are helping the world be a better place? We think so too...

Thanks for helping us help the world. You Smart Reader you...

Travis and the Smart Reads Team

WHY I STARTED SMART READS

Every time I wanted to learn about something new I'd have to buy 20 books on the topic and spend way too long sorting through them and reading them all until I arrived at the big picture. Until I had enough perspectives to know who was just guessing, who was uninformed and who had stumbled upon something remarkable.

I wished someone else could just go in and figure that out for me and tell me what matters. That's how smart reads was born. I want smart reads to be a company that does all that research up front. Sorts through all the content that is available on each topic and pulls out the most up to date complete understanding, then have people smarter than me package the best wisdom in an easy to understand way in the least amount of words possible.

For example, I got a new puppy so I wanted to learn about dog training. I bought 14 different books about dog training and by the time I got through the first 5 and finally started getting the big picture on the best way to train my puppy she had grown up into a dog.

Yeah she's well behaved. She doesn't poop in the house. I can get her to sit and come when I call. But what if someone else went in and read all those books for me, found the underlying themes and picked out the best information that would give me the big picture and get me right to the point. And I'd only have to read one book instead of 15.

That would be amazing. I would save time. And maybe my dog would be rolling over, cleaning up after my kids and doing the dishes by now. That my friend, is the reason I started smart reads. Because I wanted a company I can trust to deliver me the best information in an easy to understand way that I can digest in under an hour. Because dog training is one of many subjects I want to master.

The quicker I can learn a wide variety of topics the sooner that information can begin playing a role in shaping my future. And none of us knows how long that future will be. So why not do everything we can to make the best of it and consume a ton of knowledge. And I figured all the better if I can also make a positive difference in the world.

That's why we're also building schools, planting trees and challenging ideas about copyright's place in today's world. Because as a company we have to be doing everything we can to support the ecosystem that gives us all these beautiful places to read our books. Thanks for reading.

Travis

Customers Who Bought This Customers Who Bought This Book Also Bought

The Cannabis Pharmacy: Grow Cannabis, Make Hemp Oil and Know the Difference Between THC, CBD and the Medical Benefits of Cannabinoids

Mint As Medicine: Discover The Powerful Healing Properties of Herb in Treating Headaches, Allergies, Asthma, Clarity and Peace of Mind

The Powerful Benefits of Myrrh: Effective Myrrh Recipes For Healthy & Beauty, Oil Pulling Therapy, Creativity, Aromatherapy and Improving The Mind

Beginner Gardening: Growing Vegetables and Ornamentals Epsom Salt: Holistic Recipes for Beautiful Skin, Pain Relief and Relaxation

Growing Cannabis: How to Cultivate and Make Your Own Cannabis Garden

www.ingramcontent.com/pod-product-compliance
Lightning Source LLC
Chambersburg PA
CBHW071236240726
48654CB00009B/1081